COLE M. LETCHWORTH

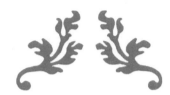

Quick & Easy Mediterranean Diet 2025

"Beginner-Friendly Recipes for Healthy, Nutritious, and Delicious Meals in Minutes; Bonus 28-Day Meal Plan to Transform Your Health"

COLE M. LETCHWORTH

BONUS; 28-Day Mediterranean-Inspired Meal Plan

Week 1

Day 1:
Breakfast: Greek Yogurt Parfait with Honey and Nuts
Lunch: Classic Greek Salad with Feta Cheese
Snack: Marinated Olives and Feta Cheese
Dinner: Grilled Lemon Herb Chicken with Couscous

Day 2:
Breakfast: Avocado and Tomato Toast with Olive Oil
Lunch: Mediterranean Tuna Salad Wraps
Snack: Herbal Iced Tea with Mint and Lemon
Dinner: Mediterranean Baked Fish with Olives and Capers

Day 3:
Breakfast: Lemon and Blueberry Overnight Oats
Lunch: Quinoa Tabbouleh with Mint and Lemon
Snack: Hummus Platter with Crudités and Pita
Dinner: Shrimp Saganaki with Feta and Tomatoes

Day 4:
Breakfast: Greek Yogurt Parfait with Honey and Nuts
Lunch: Stuffed Grape Leaves (Dolmas) with a side of Greek Salad
Snack: Freshly Squeezed Mediterranean Lemonade
Dinner: Grilled Lemon Herb Chicken with Couscous

Day 5:
Breakfast: Lemon and Blueberry Overnight Oats
Lunch: Mediterranean Tuna Salad Wraps
Snack: Marinated Olives and Feta Cheese
Dinner: Mediterranean Baked Fish with Olives and Capers

Day 6:
Breakfast: Avocado and Tomato Toast with Olive Oil
Lunch: Quinoa Tabbouleh with Mint and Lemon
Snack: Herbal Iced Tea with Mint and Lemon
Dinner: Shrimp Saganaki with Feta and Tomatoes

Day 7:
Breakfast: Greek Yogurt Parfait with Honey and Nuts
Lunch: Classic Greek Salad with Feta Cheese
Snack: Hummus Platter with Crudités and Pita
Dinner: Grilled Lemon Herb Chicken with Couscous
Dessert: Baklava with Walnuts and Honey

Week 2

Repeat Week 1 meals, but switch the order of lunch and dinner each day to add variety. Add Orange and Almond Cake as dessert on Day 14.

Week 3

Day 15:
Breakfast: Lemon and Blueberry Overnight Oats
Lunch: Mediterranean Tuna Salad Wraps
Snack: Freshly Squeezed Mediterranean Lemonade
Dinner: Mediterranean Baked Fish with Olives and Capers

Day 16:
Breakfast: Greek Yogurt Parfait with Honey and Nuts
Lunch: Quinoa Tabbouleh with Mint and Lemon
Snack: Herbal Iced Tea with Mint and Lemon
Dinner: Grilled Lemon Herb Chicken with Couscous

Day 17:
Breakfast: Avocado and Tomato Toast with Olive Oil
Lunch: Classic Greek Salad with Feta Cheese
Snack: Marinated Olives and Feta Cheese
Dinner: Shrimp Saganaki with Feta and Tomatoes

Day 18:
Breakfast: Lemon and Blueberry Overnight Oats
Lunch: Stuffed Grape Leaves (Dolmas) with a side of Greek Salad
Snack: Hummus Platter with Crudités and Pita

Dinner: Mediterranean Baked Fish with Olives and Capers

Day 19:
Breakfast: Greek Yogurt Parfait with Honey and Nuts
Lunch: Mediterranean Tuna Salad Wraps
Snack: Herbal Iced Tea with Mint and Lemon
Dinner: Grilled Lemon Herb Chicken with Couscous

Day 20:
Breakfast: Avocado and Tomato Toast with Olive Oil
Lunch: Quinoa Tabbouleh with Mint and Lemon
Snack: Freshly Squeezed Mediterranean Lemonade
Dinner: Shrimp Saganaki with Feta and Tomatoes

Day 21:
Breakfast: Lemon and Blueberry Overnight Oats
Lunch: Classic Greek Salad with Feta Cheese
Snack: Marinated Olives and Feta Cheese
Dinner: Mediterranean Baked Fish with Olives and Capers
Dessert: Greek Rice Pudding (Rizogalo)

Week 4

Repeat meals from Week 3, but add desserts and beverages creatively. On Day 28, celebrate with a complete platter of Hummus, Crudités, Stuffed Grape Leaves, and Baklava.

TABLE OF CONTENTS

Introduction

Welcome to the Mediterranean Lifestyle

The Mediterranean Diet is more than just a way of eating; it is a celebration of life, health, and community. Rooted in the traditions of countries bordering the Mediterranean Sea, this lifestyle is renowned for its emphasis on fresh, wholesome ingredients, balanced nutrition, and convivial meals shared with loved ones. Whether you are seeking to improve your health, explore new culinary horizons, or simply enjoy delicious and satisfying meals, the Mediterranean Diet offers a path that is as sustainable as it is flavorful. Welcome to a journey of vibrant tastes, timeless traditions, and healthy living.

Benefits of the Mediterranean Diet

The Mediterranean Diet has been celebrated globally for its numerous health benefits, making it one of the most recommended dietary patterns by health experts. Here are some of its key advantages:

1. **Heart Health:** Rich in healthy fats from olive oil, nuts, and fish, this diet supports cardiovascular health and reduces the risk of heart disease.

2. **Weight Management:** The emphasis on whole, unprocessed foods and portion control aids in maintaining a healthy weight.

3. **Reduced Risk of Chronic Diseases:** The diet's high content of antioxidants from fruits, vegetables, and whole grains helps lower the risk of chronic illnesses such as diabetes and certain cancers.

4. **Improved Mental Health:** Omega-3 fatty acids found in fish and nuts have been linked to improved mood and cognitive function.

5. **Longevity:** Studies have shown that adhering to a Mediterranean Diet can lead to a longer life expectancy.

6. **Anti-inflammatory Properties:** Ingredients like olive oil, tomatoes, and leafy greens help reduce inflammation in the body.

7. **Sustainability:** The focus on plant-based foods and minimal processed products supports environmental sustainability.

Embracing the Mediterranean Diet is not just a choice for better health but also a commitment to a lifestyle that promotes overall well-being and harmony with nature.

Key Ingredients and Pantry Staples

The foundation of the Mediterranean Diet is its reliance on fresh, wholesome, and nutrient-dense ingredients. Stock your pantry and fridge with these staples to bring Mediterranean flavors to your table:

Oils and Fats

- Extra virgin olive oil (the cornerstone of Mediterranean cooking)
- Olives
- Nuts and seeds (almonds, walnuts, sunflower seeds)

Grains

- Whole grains (quinoa, farro, barley, bulgur)
- Pasta (preferably whole wheat)
- Rice (such as arborio or basmati)

Legumes

- Chickpeas
- Lentils
- Beans (white beans, black beans, fava beans)

Vegetables

- Tomatoes (fresh, canned, and sun-dried)
- Eggplant
- Zucchini
- Bell peppers
- Leafy greens (spinach, kale, arugula)
- Onions and garlic

Fruits

- Citrus fruits (lemons, oranges)
- Berries (strawberries, blueberries)
- Stone fruits (peaches, apricots)
- Figs and dates

Dairy

- Yogurt (preferably Greek)
- Cheese (feta, halloumi, parmesan)

Proteins

- Fish (salmon, sardines, tuna)
- Poultry (chicken, turkey)
- Eggs

Herbs and Spices

- Fresh herbs (basil, parsley, mint, oregano, dill)
- Spices (cumin, paprika, cinnamon)

Other Essentials

- Vinegar (balsamic, red wine vinegar)
- Honey
- Capers

Having these ingredients on hand will ensure that you are always prepared to create a delicious Mediterranean-inspired meal. Together, they form the building blocks of a cuisine that is as nourishing as it is delightful.

1.

Breakfast Recipes

Greek Yogurt Parfait with Honey and Nuts

Time of Preparation

- **Preparation Time:** 10 minutes
- **Cooking Time:** None

Serving Unit

- Serves 2

Ingredients

- 2 cups Greek yogurt (plain, full-fat or low-fat as desired)
- 4 tablespoons honey
- 1/2 cup mixed nuts (almonds, walnuts, pistachios), chopped
- 1/4 cup granola (optional)
- 1/2 cup fresh berries (blueberries, strawberries, or raspberries)
- 1 teaspoon chia seeds (optional)

Procedure

1. **Prepare Ingredients:** Gather all the ingredients and ensure the nuts are roughly chopped.

2. **Layer Yogurt:** In two serving glasses or bowls, spoon a layer of Greek yogurt to cover the bottom.

3. **Add Honey and Nuts:** Drizzle a tablespoon of honey over the yogurt and sprinkle a layer of chopped nuts.

4. **Repeat Layers:** Add another layer of yogurt, followed by more honey, nuts, and granola if using.

5. **Top with Berries:** Finish with a generous topping of fresh berries and a sprinkle of chia seeds if desired.

6. **Serve Immediately:** Enjoy the parfait as a quick breakfast or a healthy dessert.

Nutritional Values (per serving)

- **Calories:** 320
- **Protein:** 14g
- **Fat:** 12g
  - Saturated Fat: 3g
- **Carbohydrates:** 35g
  - Fiber: 4g
  - Sugars: 24g
- **Calcium:** 15% of Daily Value
- **Vitamin C:** 8% of Daily Value

Cooking Tips

- For added crunch, toast the nuts lightly before using.
- Swap honey with maple syrup or agave nectar for a different flavor profile.
- Use seasonal fruits to keep the recipe fresh and exciting.
- To reduce sugar, opt for unsweetened yogurt and use less honey.

Point Value (Weight Loss-Friendly)

- Depending on your diet plan, this recipe can range between 6-8 points for most weight management programs.

Health Benefits

1. **Rich in Protein:** Greek yogurt provides high-quality protein, aiding in muscle repair and satiety.

2. **Heart-Healthy Fats:** Nuts are a great source of monounsaturated fats, which promote heart health.

3. **Antioxidants:** Fresh berries are packed with antioxidants that help combat oxidative stress.

4. **Probiotics:** Yogurt contains live cultures that support gut health and digestion.

5. **Low in Processed Sugar:** Sweetened naturally with honey and fruits, this parfait avoids refined sugars.

6. **Energy-Boosting:** The combination of protein, healthy fats, and carbohydrates makes it a perfect energy-packed meal.

Avocado and Tomato Toast with Olive Oil

Time of Preparation

- **Preparation Time:** 5 minutes
- **Cooking Time:** None

Serving Unit

- Serve 1

Ingredients

- 1 slice of whole-grain or sourdough bread
- 1/2 ripe avocado
- 1 small tomato, sliced
- 1 teaspoon extra virgin olive oil
- Pinch of sea salt
- Pinch of black pepper
- Optional: Fresh basil or microgreens for garnish

Procedure

1. **Prepare Bread:** Toast the slice of bread to your desired level of crispness.

2. **Mash Avocado:** Scoop the avocado flesh into a bowl and mash it lightly with a fork, leaving some chunks for texture.

3. **Assemble Toast:** Spread the mashed avocado onto the toasted bread evenly.

4. **Add Tomato Slices:** Lay the tomato slices over the avocado.

5. **Drizzle Olive Oil:** Drizzle extra virgin olive oil on top of the tomato slices.

6. **Season and Garnish:** Sprinkle a pinch of sea salt and black pepper. Garnish with fresh basil or microgreens if desired.

7. **Serve Immediately:** Enjoy as a light breakfast or snack.

Nutritional Values (per serving)

- **Calories:** 220

- **Protein:** 5g

- **Fat:** 15g

    o Saturated Fat: 2g

- **Carbohydrates:** 18g

    o Fiber: 7g

    o Sugars: 3g

- **Vitamin A:** 10% of Daily Value

- **Vitamin C:** 15% of Daily Value

- **Potassium:** 12% of Daily Value

Cooking Tips

- For added flavor, rub a clove of garlic on the toasted bread before spreading the avocado.

- Use heirloom tomatoes for a sweeter and more robust flavor.

- Add a pinch of red chili flakes for a slight kick.

- Sprinkle nutritional yeast for a cheesy flavor without dairy.

Point Value (Weight Loss-Friendly)

- Depending on your diet plan, this recipe is approximately 4-6 points.

Health Benefits

1. **Rich in Healthy Fats:** Avocado and olive oil provide heart-healthy monounsaturated fats.

2. **High in Fiber:** Whole-grain bread and avocado are excellent sources of dietary fiber, supporting digestion and satiety.

3. **Antioxidant-Rich:** Tomatoes offer antioxidants like lycopene, which may reduce the risk of certain chronic diseases.

4. **Supports Weight Management:** This nutrient-dense meal is satisfying yet low in calories.

5. **Promotes Skin Health:** The healthy fats and vitamins in avocado and olive oil nourish the skin.

Lemon and Blueberry Overnight Oats

Time of Preparation

- **Preparation Time:** 5 minutes
- **Cooking Time:** None (overnight refrigeration required)

Serving Unit

- Serves 2

Ingredients

- 1 cup rolled oats
- 1 cup unsweetened almond milk (or milk of choice)
- 1/2 cup Greek yogurt
- 1/2 cup fresh blueberries
- 1 tablespoon honey or maple syrup
- Zest of 1 lemon
- 1 teaspoon chia seeds
- Optional: Additional blueberries and lemon zest for topping

Procedure

1. **Combine Ingredients:** In a medium-sized bowl or two jars, mix the oats, almond milk, Greek yogurt, honey, lemon zest, and chia seeds.
2. **Add Blueberries:** Gently fold in the blueberries.
3. **Refrigerate Overnight:** Cover the bowl or jars and place them in the refrigerator for at least 6-8 hours or overnight.
4. **Serve:** In the morning, stir the oats, adjust the consistency with more milk if needed, and top with additional blueberries and lemon zest if desired.

Nutritional Values (per serving)

- **Calories:** 250
- **Protein:** 9g
- **Fat:** 6g
    - Saturated Fat: 1g
- **Carbohydrates:** 40g
    - Fiber: 7g
    - Sugars: 10g
- **Vitamin C:** 12% of Daily Value
- **Calcium:** 15% of Daily Value

Cooking Tips

- Use steel-cut oats for a chewier texture but increase the liquid slightly.
- Swap blueberries with raspberries, strawberries, or blackberries for variety.
- Add a pinch of cinnamon or vanilla extract for enhanced flavor.
- For added crunch, sprinkle toasted nuts or granola before serving.

Point Value (Weight Loss-Friendly)

- This recipe typically falls within 5-7 points for most weight management programs.

Health Benefits

1. **Supports Digestion:** Chia seeds and oats are excellent sources of fiber, promoting digestive health.

2. **Boosts Immunity:** Blueberries provide antioxidants and vitamin C, which support immune function.

3. **Heart-Healthy:** The combination of oats and blueberries contributes to cardiovascular health.

4. **Sustains Energy:** The balanced macronutrients ensure a steady release of energy throughout the day.

5. **Promotes Bone Health:** Greek yogurt and almond milk are good sources of calcium.

2.

Lunch Recipes

Classic Greek Salad with Feta Cheese

Preparation Time: 10 minutes
Cooking Time: None
Serving Unit: Serves 4

Ingredients:

- 1 large cucumber, sliced
- 2-3 medium tomatoes, chopped
- 1 red onion, thinly sliced
- 1 bell pepper (any color), chopped
- 1 cup Kalamata olives, pitted
- 200g feta cheese, cubed or in large block
- 2-3 tablespoons extra virgin olive oil
- 1 tablespoon red wine vinegar
- 1 teaspoon dried oregano
- Salt and freshly ground black pepper to taste
- Optional: Fresh parsley or basil for garnish

Procedure:

1. **Prepare the vegetables:** Slice the cucumber, tomatoes, onion, and bell pepper into bite-sized pieces.

2. **Assemble the salad:** In a large bowl, combine the cucumber, tomatoes, onion, bell pepper, and Kalamata olives. Toss gently to mix.

3. **Add the feta:** Either crumble the feta into the salad or cut it into cubes or a large block, depending on your preference.

4. **Dress the salad:** Drizzle olive oil and red wine vinegar over the ingredients. Sprinkle with dried oregano, salt, and pepper.

5. **Toss and serve:** Give the salad a gentle toss to coat the ingredients evenly with the dressing. Garnish with fresh herbs if desired.

Nutritional Values (per serving):

- **Calories:** 250 kcal
- **Protein:** 6g
- **Fat:** 21g (of which saturated fat is 7g)
- **Carbohydrates:** 10g
- **Fiber:** 2g
- **Sugar:** 4g
- **Sodium:** 650mg

Cooking Tips:

- For the best flavor, allow the salad to sit for a few minutes after tossing, so the flavors can meld together.

- Use good-quality extra virgin olive oil and high-quality feta for the best taste.

- You can substitute the feta with a plant-based version if you are looking for a vegan option.

- Add a sprinkle of toasted pine nuts for extra texture and flavor.

Point Value:

- **Weight Watchers Smart Points:** Approximately 6 points per serving.

Health Benefits:

- **Rich in antioxidants:** The tomatoes, bell peppers, and olives provide a great source of antioxidants like vitamin C and lycopene, which can help fight inflammation and promote heart health.

- **Good for bone health:** Feta cheese is a good source of calcium, which supports bone health.

- **Healthy fats:** The olive oil in this recipe is rich in monounsaturated fats, which are heart-healthy and can improve cholesterol levels.

- **Low in calories:** This salad is low in calories while being nutrient-dense, making it an ideal choice for weight management.

Quinoa Tabbouleh with Mint and Lemon

Preparation Time: 15 minutes
Cooking Time: 15 minutes
Serving Unit: Serves 4

Ingredients:

- 1 cup quinoa (uncooked)
- 2 medium tomatoes, diced
- 1 cucumber, diced
- 1 small red onion, finely chopped
- 1/4 cup fresh parsley, chopped
- 1/4 cup fresh mint, chopped
- Juice of 2 lemons
- 2 tablespoons extra virgin olive oil
- Salt and freshly ground black pepper to taste
- Optional: 1 tablespoon pomegranate seeds for garnish

Procedure:

1. **Cook the quinoa:** Rinse the quinoa under cold water to remove its bitter coating. In a saucepan, add 2 cups of water for 1 cup of quinoa, bring to a boil, then reduce the heat to low and simmer, covered, for about 15 minutes or until the water is absorbed and the quinoa is tender. Let it cool to room temperature.

2. **Prepare the vegetables and herbs:** While the quinoa is cooking, chop the tomatoes, cucumber, red onion, parsley, and mint.

3. **Combine the ingredients:** In a large bowl, combine the cooled quinoa with the diced vegetables and herbs.

4. **Dress the salad:** Add the lemon juice, olive oil, salt, and pepper to the quinoa mixture. Stir gently to combine.

5. **Garnish and serve:** Optionally, garnish with pomegranate seeds for an added burst of color and flavor. Serve chilled or at room temperature.

Nutritional Values (per serving):

- **Calories:** 220 kcal

- **Protein:** 6g

- **Fat:** 9g (of which 1g is saturated fat)

- **Carbohydrates:** 30g

- **Fiber:** 5g

- **Sugar:** 4g

- **Sodium:** 45mg

Cooking Tips:

- Rinse the quinoa thoroughly before cooking to remove its saponin coating, which can make it taste bitter.

- For a more filling dish, add some chickpeas or grilled chicken for extra protein.

- Let the salad sit in the fridge for an hour before serving to allow the flavors to meld together.

- This dish is versatile—feel free to add other herbs like basil or cilantro for variation.

Point Value:

- **Weight Watchers Smart Points:** Approximately 5 points per serving.

Health Benefits:

- **High in fiber:** Quinoa is a whole grain, rich in dietary fiber, which aids digestion and helps maintain stable blood sugar levels.

- **Rich in vitamins and minerals:** The fresh herbs and vegetables provide essential nutrients, including vitamin C and potassium.

- **Protein-packed:** Quinoa is a complete protein, meaning it contains all nine essential amino acids, making it an excellent plant-based protein source.

- **Anti-inflammatory:** The combination of lemon, parsley, and mint has anti-inflammatory properties, helping to reduce inflammation in the body.

Mediterranean Tuna Salad Wraps

Preparation Time: 10 minutes
Cooking Time: None
Serving Unit: Serves 4

Ingredients:

- 2 cans (5 oz each) of tuna in olive oil, drained
- 1/2 cup Greek yogurt (or mayonnaise)
- 1 tablespoon Dijon mustard
- 1 tablespoon red wine vinegar
- 1/4 cup red onion, finely chopped
- 1/2 cup cucumber, diced
- 1/4 cup Kalamata olives, chopped
- 1 tablespoon capers, drained
- 2 teaspoons dried oregano
- 4 whole wheat or spinach wraps
- Salt and freshly ground black pepper to taste
- Optional: Fresh arugula or spinach for garnish

Procedure:

1. **Prepare the tuna mixture:** In a medium bowl, combine the drained tuna, Greek yogurt, Dijon mustard, red wine vinegar, and dried oregano. Stir well to combine.

2. **Add the vegetables and olives:** Fold in the chopped red onion, cucumber, olives, and capers. Season with salt and pepper to taste.

3. **Assemble the wraps:** Lay the wraps flat on a clean surface. Spoon an equal amount of the tuna salad mixture onto the center of each wrap.

4. **Add greens and roll:** Optionally, add fresh arugula or spinach on top of the tuna mixture for added texture and nutrition. Roll the wraps tightly, folding in the sides as you go.

5. **Serve:** Cut the wraps in half and serve immediately or wrap in foil for an on-the-go meal.

Nutritional Values (per serving):

- **Calories:** 320 kcal
- **Protein:** 28g
- **Fat:** 18g (of which saturated fat is 2g)
- **Carbohydrates:** 20g
- **Fiber:** 4g
- **Sugar:** 3g
- **Sodium:** 650mg

Cooking Tips:

- For a lighter version, swap the Greek yogurt for a lower-fat variety or use a plant-based yogurt.
- You can use fresh tuna (grilled or seared) instead of canned tuna for an even more elevated dish.
- Add some diced avocado for a creamier texture and extra healthy fats.
- Make these wraps in advance and wrap them tightly in plastic wrap for a packed lunch option.

Point Value:

- **Weight Watchers Smart Points:** Approximately 7 points per serving.

Health Benefits:

- **High in protein:** Tuna is an excellent source of lean protein, which helps in muscle repair and supports immune function.

- **Heart-healthy fats:** Olive oil and tuna are both rich in omega-3 fatty acids, which are beneficial for cardiovascular health.

- **Gut-friendly:** Greek yogurt adds probiotics to the recipe, which are beneficial for gut health and digestion.

- **Low in carbohydrates:** These wraps provide a lower-carb option for those managing blood sugar or following a low-carb diet.

These **recipes** are all versatile, nutrient-dense, and quick to prepare, making them ideal for busy individuals looking for healthy meal options that don't compromise on flavor

3.

Dinner Recipes

Grilled Lemon Herb Chicken with Couscous

Preparation Time: 15 minutes
Cooking Time: 25 minutes
Serving Unit: Serves 4

Ingredients

For the Chicken Marinade:

- 4 boneless, skinless chicken breasts (about 1.5 lbs)
- 3 tablespoons olive oil
- Juice and zest of 2 lemons
- 3 cloves garlic, minced
- 1 tablespoon dried oregano
- 1 tablespoon fresh parsley, chopped
- 1 teaspoon salt
- ½ teaspoon freshly ground black pepper
- ½ teaspoon red pepper flakes (optional)

For the Couscous:

- 1 cup couscous
- 1 ¼ cups water or chicken broth
- 1 tablespoon olive oil
- 1 teaspoon salt
- Fresh parsley or cilantro, for garnish (optional)

Procedure:

1. **Marinate the chicken:** In a bowl, combine olive oil, lemon juice, lemon zest, minced garlic, dried oregano, parsley, salt, pepper, and red pepper flakes. Mix well. Place the chicken breasts in a resealable plastic bag or shallow dish and pour the marinade over. Seal and refrigerate for at least 30 minutes, or up to 4 hours for a more intense flavor.

2. **Prepare the couscous:** In a medium saucepan, bring 1 ¼ cups of water or chicken broth to a boil. Stir in the couscous, olive oil, and salt. Remove from heat and cover with a lid. Let it sit for 5 minutes, then fluff the couscous with a fork. Garnish with fresh parsley or cilantro.

3. **Grill the chicken:** Preheat a grill or grill pan to medium-high heat. Remove the chicken from the marinade and grill for about 6-7 minutes per side, or until the internal temperature reaches 165°F (74°C) and the juices run clear.

4. **Serve:** Plate the grilled chicken on a bed of couscous, drizzle with any leftover marinade (optional), and garnish with extra herbs. Serve immediately.

Nutritional Values (per serving):

- Calories: 350 kcal
- Protein: 38g
- Fat: 14g (of which 2g is saturated fat)
- Carbohydrates: 25g
- Fiber: 2g

- Sugar: 2g
- Sodium: 500mg

Cooking Tips:

- Marinate the chicken for longer if possible to enhance the flavor, as the lemon and herbs will tenderize the meat.

- If you don't have a grill, this recipe can also be made using a grill pan or baked in the oven at 375°F (190°C) for about 25 minutes.

- For extra flavor, try adding pine nuts or roasted vegetables (like bell peppers or zucchini) to the couscous.

Point Value:

- **Weight Watchers Smart Points:** Approximately 7 points per serving (without garnish).

Health Benefits:

- **Lean protein:** Chicken breast is an excellent source of lean protein, which supports muscle building and repair.

- **Rich in antioxidants:** Lemon and garlic have antioxidant properties that support immune function and reduce inflammation.

- **Good fats:** Olive oil provides heart-healthy monounsaturated fats.

- **Whole grain couscous:** The couscous provides complex carbohydrates and fiber, which help regulate blood sugar and improve digestion.

Shrimp Saganaki with Feta and Tomatoes

Preparation Time: 10 minutes
Cooking Time: 15 minutes
Serving Unit: Serves 4

Ingredients:

- 1 lb large shrimp, peeled and deveined
- 2 tablespoons olive oil
- 1 medium onion, finely chopped
- 2 cloves garlic, minced
- 1 can (14.5 oz) diced tomatoes (or 2 large fresh tomatoes, diced)
- 1 teaspoon dried oregano
- ½ teaspoon red pepper flakes (optional)
- 1 cup feta cheese, crumbled
- 1/4 cup Kalamata olives, pitted and chopped
- 1 tablespoon fresh parsley, chopped
- Salt and pepper to taste
- Lemon wedges for serving
- Fresh pita or crusty bread for dipping (optional)

Procedure:

1. **Prepare the shrimp:** Season the shrimp with salt, pepper, and 1 teaspoon of oregano.

2. **Cook the base sauce:** Heat olive oil in a large skillet over medium heat. Add the chopped onion and cook for about 5 minutes until softened and

translucent. Add the garlic and cook for another 1 minute until fragrant.

3. **Add the tomatoes:** Pour in the diced tomatoes (with their juice) and red pepper flakes (if using). Bring the mixture to a simmer and let it cook for 5-7 minutes, allowing the sauce to thicken slightly.

4. **Cook the shrimp:** Add the shrimp to the skillet and cook for 3-4 minutes, or until they are pink and opaque. Stir occasionally to ensure even cooking.

5. **Add feta and olives:** Crumble the feta cheese over the shrimp and sprinkle with Kalamata olives. Let the feta warm through and soften slightly, about 2 minutes.

6. **Serve:** Garnish with fresh parsley and serve immediately with lemon wedges and pita or crusty bread for dipping.

Nutritional Values (per serving):

- Calories: 320 kcal
- Protein: 30g
- Fat: 22g (of which 8g is saturated fat)
- Carbohydrates: 8g
- Fiber: 2g
- Sugar: 4g
- Sodium: 750mg

Cooking Tips:

- For extra flavor, marinate the shrimp in olive oil, lemon juice, garlic, and oregano for 15-20 minutes before cooking.

- This dish can be served over rice, quinoa, or couscous for a heartier meal.

- If you prefer a less salty dish, be sure to use low-sodium feta cheese and rinse the Kalamata olives before using them.

Point Value

- **Weight Watchers Smart Points:** Approximately 8 points per serving.

Health Benefits

- **High in protein:** Shrimp is a great source of lean protein, important for muscle repair and maintenance.

- **Heart-healthy fats:** The olive oil and feta provide monounsaturated fats that are beneficial for heart health.

- **Rich in antioxidants:** Tomatoes, garlic, and oregano offer antioxidants that support the immune system and reduce oxidative stress.

- **Low in carbohydrates:** This dish is ideal for low-carb or ketogenic diets.

Mediterranean Baked Fish with Olives and Capers

Preparation Time: 10 minutes
Cooking Time: 20 minutes
Serving Unit: Serves 4

Ingredients:

- 4 white fish fillets (such as cod, halibut, or tilapia)
- 2 tablespoons olive oil
- 1 lemon, thinly sliced
- 1/4 cup Kalamata olives, pitted and chopped
- 2 tablespoons capers, drained
- 1 tablespoon fresh parsley, chopped
- 1 teaspoon dried oregano
- 1/2 teaspoon garlic powder
- Salt and pepper to taste

Procedure:

1. Preheat the oven: Preheat your oven to 375°F (190°C). Lightly grease a baking dish with olive oil or line it with parchment paper.

2. Prepare the fish fillets: Season the fish fillets with salt, pepper, garlic powder, and dried oregano on both sides. Place the fillets in the prepared baking dish.

3. Add the toppings: Drizzle olive oil over the fish fillets. Top with lemon slices, chopped Kalamata olives, and capers.

4. Bake the fish: Bake the fish in the preheated oven for 15-20 minutes, or until the fish is opaque and flakes easily with a fork. The cooking time will depend on the thickness of the fillets.

5. Serve: Remove from the oven and garnish with fresh parsley. Serve with roasted vegetables or a light salad for a complete meal.

Nutritional Values (per serving):

- Calories: 220 kcal
- Protein: 26g
- Fat: 12g (of which 2g is saturated fat)
- Carbohydrates: 3g
- Fiber: 1g
- Sugar: 1g
- Sodium: 850mg

Cooking Tips:

- If using a thicker fish fillet (like halibut), check for doneness by inserting a fork into the thickest part of the fish; it should flake easily.
- For added flavor, drizzle a little extra lemon juice on the fish just before serving.
- Serve this dish with a side of quinoa or couscous for a complete Mediterranean meal.

Point Value:

- Weight Watchers SmartPoints: Approximately 4 points per serving.

Health Benefits:

- Rich in omega-3 fatty acids: The fish provides a healthy dose of omega-3s, which are essential for heart health and reducing inflammation.

- Low in calories: This dish is low in calories, making it a great option for those watching their weight.

- High in protein: The fish is an excellent source of high-quality protein, supporting muscle maintenance and overall health.

- Rich in antioxidants: Olives, capers, and lemon provide antioxidants that help protect the body from oxidative stress and support immune function.

These Mediterranean-inspired recipes offer a variety of flavors and nutrients that are beneficial for overall health. They're simple, quick to prepare, and versatile enough for a variety of dietary preferences, making them great options for busy weeknights or weekend gatherings

4.

Snacks and Appetizers

Hummus Platter with Crudités and Pita

Preparation Time: 15 minutes
Cooking Time: None
Serving Unit: Serves 4

Ingredients:

For the Hummus (store-bought or homemade):

- 1 can (15 oz) chickpeas, drained and rinsed (or 1.5 cups cooked chickpeas)
- 1/4 cup tahini
- 2 tablespoons olive oil
- 2 tablespoons fresh lemon juice
- 1-2 cloves garlic, minced
- 1/2 teaspoon ground cumin
- Salt to taste
- Water (as needed for consistency)
- 1 tablespoon paprika or sumac (for garnish)
- Fresh parsley (optional, for garnish)

For the Crudités (vegetable dipping platter):

- 1 cucumber, sliced into rounds
- 2-3 carrots, cut into sticks
- 1 bell pepper, cut into strips
- 1 cup cherry tomatoes, halved
- 1/2 cup celery sticks

For the Pita:

- 4-6 pita bread rounds, cut into wedges
- 1 tablespoon olive oil (optional, for brushing on pita)

Procedure:

1. **Prepare the hummus:**
   If making homemade hummus, combine the chickpeas, tahini, olive oil, lemon juice, garlic, cumin, and salt in a food processor. Blend until smooth, adding water as needed to reach your desired consistency. Taste and adjust seasoning as needed.

2. **Prepare the vegetables:**
   Arrange the cucumber, carrot sticks, bell pepper strips, cherry tomatoes, and celery on a large platter, keeping the vegetables separate for a variety of dipping options.

3. **Prepare the pita:**
   If you want warm, crisp pita wedges, preheat your oven to 350°F (175°C). Brush the pita bread with olive oil and cut it into wedges. Place the wedges on a baking sheet and bake for 8-10 minutes until lightly golden and crispy.

4. **Assemble the platter:**
   Place the hummus in a bowl at the center of the platter. Arrange the crudités and pita wedges around the hummus. Garnish the hummus with a sprinkle of paprika or sumac and a few sprigs of fresh parsley, if desired.

5. **Serve:**
   Serve immediately as an appetizer or snack. Enjoy the freshness of the

veggies and the creamy hummus with the warm pita.

Nutritional Values (per serving):

- **Calories:** 250 kcal

- **Protein:** 7g

- **Fat:** 14g (of which 2g is saturated fat)

- **Carbohydrates:** 30g

- **Fiber:** 8g

- **Sugar:** 5g

- **Sodium:** 330mg

Cooking Tips:

- For extra creaminess in your hummus, peel the skins off the chickpeas before blending. This is a little tedious but results in a smoother texture.

- Add more lemon juice or garlic depending on your personal preference.

- To make the pita wedges extra crispy, try brushing them with a bit of garlic-infused olive oil before baking.

- For a variation, add roasted red peppers or olives to the hummus for a different flavor profile.

Point Value:

- **Weight Watchers Smart Points:** Approximately 6 points per serving (without pita).

Health Benefits:

- **High in fiber:** Hummus and the accompanying vegetables are rich in dietary fiber, which aids digestion, helps maintain stable blood sugar, and supports heart health.

- **Rich in healthy fats:** Olive oil and tahini provide monounsaturated fats, which are beneficial for heart health.

- **Plant-based protein:** Chickpeas offer plant-based protein, important for muscle repair and general body function.

- **Antioxidants:** Vegetables like bell peppers and tomatoes are rich in vitamins A and C, which support immune function and skin health.

Stuffed Grape Leaves (Dolmas)

Preparation Time: 30 minutes
Cooking Time: 40 minutes
Serving Unit: Serves 6

Ingredients:

For the Filling:

- 1 cup short-grain rice (such as Arborio or Basmati)
- 1/2 cup onion, finely chopped
- 2 tablespoons olive oil
- 1 teaspoon ground cumin
- 1 teaspoon ground coriander
- 1/2 teaspoon cinnamon
- 1/4 teaspoon allspice
- 2 tablespoons fresh dill, chopped
- 1 tablespoon fresh parsley, chopped
- Juice of 1 lemon
- Salt and pepper to taste

For the Dolmas:

- 1 jar (about 16 oz) grape leaves in brine, drained and rinsed
- 1/4 cup olive oil (for drizzling)
- 1-2 cups water (for steaming)

Procedure:

1. **Prepare the filling:**
   In a pan, heat olive oil over medium heat. Add the chopped onion and cook until soft and translucent, about 5 minutes. Add the rice and cook for another 2 minutes, stirring occasionally. Add cumin, coriander, cinnamon, and allspice, and cook for 1 minute until fragrant. Stir in the fresh dill, parsley, lemon juice, salt, and pepper. Remove from heat and let it cool.

2. **Stuff the grape leaves:**
   Lay a grape leaf flat on a work surface with the vein side facing up. Place about 1 tablespoon of the rice filling near the stem end of the leaf. Fold in the sides of the leaf and roll tightly from the bottom up to form a small, tight package. Repeat with the remaining leaves and filling.

3. **Cook the dolmas:**
   Arrange the stuffed grape leaves seam side down in a large pot. Pour olive oil over the dolmas and add enough water to cover them. Place a plate on top of the dolmas to keep them submerged. Bring the water to a simmer over medium heat, then cover and cook for about 40 minutes, or until the rice is fully cooked and tender.

4. **Serve:**
   Let the dolmas cool slightly before serving. They are often served with a side of plain yogurt or a drizzle of fresh lemon juice.

Nutritional Values (per serving):

- **Calories:** 180 kcal
- **Protein:** 4g
- **Fat:** 9g (of which 1g is saturated fat)

23

- **Carbohydrates:** 25g

- **Fiber:** 5g

- **Sugar:** 1g

- **Sodium:** 330mg

Cooking Tips:

- If you can't find jarred grape leaves, you can blanch fresh grape leaves in boiling water for 2-3 minutes to soften them.

- The filling can be varied with ground lamb or beef if you want a heartier option.

- If you find grape leaves too salty, soak them in warm water for 30 minutes before using them.

- Dolmas can be served at room temperature or chilled for a refreshing appetizer.

Point Value:

- Weight Watchers SmartPoints: Approximately 4 points per serving.

Health Benefits:

- Rich in fiber: The rice and grape leaves provide a good amount of fiber, which supports digestive health and helps maintain blood sugar levels.

- Low in calories: Dolmas are low in calories, making them an excellent snack or appetizer for those managing their weight.

- Herbs and spices: Dill, parsley, and other spices add antioxidants and anti-inflammatory compounds that contribute to overall well-being.

- Plant-based: These dolmas are plant-based, making them suitable for vegetarians or those following a plant-based diet.

Marinated Olives and Feta Cheese

Preparation Time: 10 minutes
Cooking Time: None
Serving Unit: Serves 4

Ingredients:

- 1 1/2 cups mixed olives (green, Kalamata, and black)
- 1/2 cup feta cheese, cubed
- 2 tablespoons olive oil
- 1 tablespoon red wine vinegar
- 1 teaspoon dried oregano
- 1/2 teaspoon red pepper flakes
- 1 clove garlic, minced
- Zest of 1 lemon
- Fresh parsley for garnish

Procedure:

1. **Prepare the marinade:**
   In a bowl, combine the olive oil, red wine vinegar, oregano, red pepper flakes, garlic, and lemon zest. Stir to combine.

2. **Marinate the olives and feta:**
   Add the olives and feta cheese to the marinade. Toss gently to coat the olives and cheese evenly with the marinade. Let the mixture sit for at least 30 minutes at room temperature (or refrigerate for up to 2-3 hours for more intense flavor).

3. **Serve:**
   Before serving, give the olives and feta a quick stir and garnish with fresh parsley. Serve as an appetizer with crusty bread or alongside a Mediterranean platter.

Nutritional Values (per serving):

- **Calories:** 200 kcal
- **Protein:** 6g
- **Fat:** 18g (of which 5g is saturated fat)
- **Carbohydrates:** 6g
- **Fiber:** 2g
- **Sugar:** 1g
- **Sodium:** 900mg

Cooking Tips:

- If you're using store-bought feta, you can rinse it briefly to reduce the salt content before marinating.

- For a more vibrant flavor, add a few slices of lemon or orange to the marinade.

- These marinated olives and feta can be served as part of a mezze platter or as a quick appetizer for a Mediterranean meal.

Point Value:

- **Weight Watchers Smart Points:** Approximately 6 points per serving.

Health Benefits:

- **Heart-healthy fats:** The olives and olive oil provide monounsaturated fats, which support cardiovascular health.

- **Rich in calcium:** Feta cheese is a good source of calcium, which is essential for bone health.

- **Antioxidants:** Olives and herbs like oregano are rich in antioxidants, which help protect the body from oxidative stress and inflammation.

- **Low in carbohydrates:** This dish is ideal for low-carb or ketogenic diets.

These Mediterranean-inspired recipes offer vibrant, healthy, and flavorful options that make for satisfying snacks, appetizers, or light meals. They are easy to prepare, packed with nutrients, and a great way to incorporate the wholesome ingredients of the Mediterranean diet into your meals.

5.

Desserts

Baklava with Walnuts and Honey

Preparation Time: 30 minutes
Cooking Time: 45 minutes
Serving Unit: Serves 8-10

Ingredients:

For the Baklava:

- 1 package (16 oz) phyllo dough, thawed

- 2 cups walnuts, finely chopped (or mixed nuts, if desired)

- 1 teaspoon ground cinnamon

- 1 cup unsalted butter, melted

- 1 cup granulated sugar

- 1 cup water

- 1/2 cup honey

- 1 teaspoon vanilla extract

- 1 teaspoon lemon juice

Procedure:

1. **Prepare the nut filling:**
   In a bowl, combine the chopped walnuts and ground cinnamon. Set aside.

2. **Prepare the baking dish:**
   Preheat your oven to 350°F (175°C). Brush a 9x13-inch baking dish with some of the melted butter.

3. **Assemble the baklava:**
   Place one sheet of phyllo dough in the baking dish and brush it generously with melted butter. Repeat this step, layering and buttering each sheet, for about 8-10 sheets. After 10 layers, sprinkle a thin layer of the walnut-cinnamon mixture evenly over the phyllo.

Continue layering phyllo sheets and buttering them, followed by a layer of nuts. Repeat this process until all the nuts are used up, and then finish by layering the remaining phyllo sheets, again buttering each one. You should have about 20-25 layers of phyllo in total.

4. **Cut the baklava:**
   Before baking, use a sharp knife to cut the baklava into diamond or square shapes. This will help it cook evenly and make it easier to serve.

5. **Bake the baklava:**
   Bake the baklava in the preheated oven for 40-45 minutes, or until the phyllo is golden brown and crisp.

6. **Prepare the syrup:**
   While the baklava is baking, make the syrup. In a saucepan, combine the granulated sugar, water, honey, vanilla extract, and lemon juice. Bring to a boil over medium heat, then lower the heat and let it simmer for about 10-15 minutes until the syrup thickens slightly.

7. **Pour the syrup over the baklava:**
   Once the baklava is done baking, remove it from the oven and immediately pour the hot syrup over the crispy layers. Let the baklava sit at room temperature for several hours or overnight to absorb the

syrup and become perfectly sweet and sticky.

8. **Serve:**
Serve the baklava at room temperature. It will keep for up to a week if stored in an airtight container.

Nutritional Values (per serving):

- **Calories:** 350 kcal

- **Protein:** 4g

- **Fat:** 21g (of which 5g is saturated fat)

- **Carbohydrates:** 40g

- **Fiber:** 2g

- **Sugar:** 30g

- **Sodium:** 45mg

Cooking Tips:

- Be sure to brush each layer of phyllo with enough butter to ensure it crisps up properly in the oven.

- You can experiment with different nuts, such as pistachios, almonds, or pecans, for varied flavors.

- If you want to make your baklava extra indulgent, you can drizzle a bit of melted chocolate over the top once it has cooled.

- Baklava can be stored at room temperature in an airtight container for up to a week, but the syrupy layers tend to soften over time.

Point Value:

- **Weight Watchers Smart Points:** Approximately 12 points per serving.

Health Benefits:

- **Good source of healthy fats:** Walnuts provide heart-healthy omega-3 fatty acids.

- **Rich in antioxidants:** Honey and walnuts are packed with antioxidants that help reduce inflammation and support overall health.

- **Moderate sugar content:** While baklava is high in sugar, consuming it in moderation as part of a balanced diet can still be a satisfying treat without overindulging.

Orange and Almond Cake

Preparation Time: 20 minutes
Cooking Time: 45 minutes
Serving Unit: Serves 8

Ingredients:

For the Cake:

- 1 1/2 cups almond meal (or finely ground almonds)
- 1 cup granulated sugar
- 4 large eggs
- 1/2 cup unsalted butter, softened
- 1/4 cup fresh orange juice
- Zest of 2 oranges
- 1 teaspoon vanilla extract
- 1 teaspoon baking powder
- Pinch of salt

For the Glaze:

- 1/4 cup fresh orange juice
- 2 tablespoons powdered sugar

Procedure:

1. **Preheat the oven:**
   Preheat your oven to 350°F (175°C). Grease and line a 9-inch round cake pan with parchment paper.

2. **Prepare the cake batter:**
   In a large bowl, beat the softened butter and sugar together until light and fluffy. Add the eggs, one at a time, beating well after each addition. Mix in the orange juice, orange zest, and vanilla extract.

3. **Add dry ingredients:**
   In a separate bowl, combine the almond meal, baking powder, and salt. Gradually add this mixture to the wet ingredients, stirring until fully incorporated. The batter will be thick but smooth.

4. **Bake the cake:**
   Pour the batter into the prepared cake pan and smooth the top. Bake for 40-45 minutes, or until the cake is golden brown and a toothpick inserted into the center comes out clean.

5. **Prepare the glaze:**
   While the cake is baking, whisk together the fresh orange juice and powdered sugar in a small bowl until smooth. Set aside.

6. **Finish the cake:**
   Once the cake has cooled slightly, drizzle the orange glaze over the top of the cake. Let it set for a few minutes before slicing and serving.

7. **Serve:**
   Slice the cake into wedges and serve at room temperature. It pairs wonderfully with a cup of tea or coffee.

Nutritional Values (per serving):

- **Calories:** 280 kcal
- **Protein:** 6g
- **Fat:** 20g (of which 3g is saturated fat)

- **Carbohydrates:** 25g
- **Fiber:** 3g
- **Sugar:** 15g
- **Sodium:** 100mg

Cooking Tips:

- If you don't have almond meal, you can grind whole almonds in a food processor until finely ground.

- For added flavor, try sprinkling some sliced almonds on top of the cake before baking.

- This cake is naturally gluten-free because it uses almond meal instead of wheat flour.

- The glaze can be adjusted to your sweetness preference—add more powdered sugar if you want it sweeter, or less for a more subtle finish.

Point Value:

- **Weight Watchers Smart Points:** Approximately 9 points per serving.

Health Benefits:

- **Almonds are heart-healthy:** Rich in monounsaturated fats, almonds can help improve cholesterol levels and promote heart health.

- **Vitamin C from oranges:** The fresh orange juice and zest provide vitamin C, an essential antioxidant for immune function.

- **Gluten-free:** This cake is a great option for those with gluten sensitivities or those following a gluten-free diet.

- **Good source of protein:** Almonds also provide a good amount of protein, which is important for muscle repair and overall health.

Greek Rice Pudding (Rizogalo)

Preparation Time: 10 minutes
Cooking Time: 40 minutes
Serving Unit: Serves 4-6

Ingredients:

- 1/2 cup short-grain rice (such as Arborio)

- 4 cups whole milk

- 1/2 cup granulated sugar

- 1 teaspoon vanilla extract

- 1/4 teaspoon ground cinnamon (for garnish)

- 1 tablespoon cornstarch (optional, for a thicker pudding)

Procedure:

1. **Cook the rice:**
   In a medium saucepan, combine the rice and 1 cup of water. Bring it to a boil over medium heat, then reduce the heat and simmer for about 10 minutes until the rice has absorbed most of the water.

2. **Prepare the pudding base:**
   Add the milk and sugar to the rice. Bring the mixture to a simmer over medium heat, stirring constantly. Reduce the heat to low and cook for about 25-30 minutes, stirring frequently, until the rice is soft and the mixture has thickened to a creamy consistency.

3. **Optional thickening (cornstarch):**
   If you prefer a thicker pudding, dissolve the cornstarch in a small amount of cold milk (about 1/4 cup) and stir it into the rice mixture. Cook for an additional 5 minutes, stirring until the pudding thickens.

4. **Add flavor:**
   Stir in the vanilla extract and remove the pudding from the heat. Let it cool slightly before serving.

5. **Serve:**
   Spoon the pudding into individual bowls and sprinkle with ground cinnamon on top. Serve warm or chilled, depending on your preference.

Nutritional Values (per serving):

- **Calories:** 250 kcal

- **Protein:** 6g

- **Fat:** 8g (of which 5g is saturated fat)

- **Carbohydrates:** 38g

- **Fiber:** 1g

- **Sugar:** 25g

- **Sodium:** 80mg

Cooking Tips:

- Stir the pudding constantly to prevent the rice from sticking to the bottom of the pot.

- You can make this pudding the day before and store it in the refrigerator. It will thicken further as it cools.

- For a different flavor profile, you can infuse the milk with a cinnamon stick or a strip of lemon peel while cooking, then remove them before serving.

Point Value:

- **Weight Watchers Smart Points:** Approximately 7 points per serving.

Health Benefits:

- **Good source of calcium:** The milk provides calcium, which is essential for strong bones and teeth.

- **Easily digestible:** This pudding is easy on the stomach, making it a good option for those who need a gentle dessert.

- **Satisfying comfort food:** Rizogalo is a warm and comforting treat, ideal for cooling evenings or when you're in need of a light yet satisfying dessert.

These Mediterranean-inspired desserts offer a delightful mix of textures and flavors, from the crispy, sweet layers of baklava to the citrusy richness of the orange almond cake and the creamy comfort of rice pudding. Perfect for rounding off a meal or serving at a special gathering, each dish also provides nutritional benefits, making them more than just a treat!

6.

Beverages

Herbal Iced Tea with Mint and Lemon

Preparation Time: 5 minutes
Infusion Time: 10 minutes
Chill Time: 1-2 hours
Serving Unit: Serves 4-6

Ingredients:

- 4-6 herbal tea bags (e.g., chamomile, green tea, or lemon balm)
- 4 cups boiling water
- 1/4 cup fresh mint leaves, roughly chopped
- 2 tablespoons honey or agave syrup (optional, adjust to taste)
- 1 lemon, thinly sliced
- Ice cubes
- Fresh mint sprigs, for garnish (optional)

Procedure:

1. **Brew the tea:**
   In a heatproof pitcher, place the herbal tea bags. Pour the boiling water over the tea bags and allow them to steep for 5-7 minutes, depending on the strength you desire. After steeping, remove the tea bags and discard them.

2. **Add fresh mint and lemon:**
   While the tea is still warm, add the fresh mint leaves and honey (or agave syrup) if you're using it. Stir gently to combine. The warmth of the tea will help release the mint's flavor and dissolve the sweetener. Add the lemon slices to infuse the tea with a citrusy brightness.

3. **Cool and chill:**
   Allow the tea to cool to room temperature, then transfer the pitcher to the refrigerator to chill for 1-2 hours, or until it's cold and refreshing.

4. **Serve:**
   To serve, fill glasses with ice cubes and pour the chilled tea over the ice. Garnish with additional mint sprigs or lemon slices if desired.

5. **Enjoy:**
   Refresh yourself with this invigorating herbal iced tea, perfect for hot days or as a revitalizing drink to accompany any meal.

Nutritional Values (per serving):

- **Calories:** 5-15 kcal (depending on sweetener choice)
- **Protein:** 0g
- **Fat:** 0g
- **Carbohydrates:** 1-3g (from honey/agave)
- **Fiber:** 0g
- **Sugar:** 1-3g (from honey/agave)
- **Sodium:** 5mg

Cooking Tips:

- **Adjust sweetness:** Feel free to adjust the sweetness based on your preference. If you prefer a more natural sweetener, consider using stevia or maple syrup.

- **Herb variation:** You can add a sprig of rosemary or basil for a unique twist on the traditional mint flavor.

- **Tea bags:** If you're using stronger herbal tea like green tea, reduce the steeping time to avoid bitterness.

- **Ice cubes:** For an extra refreshing touch, freeze some mint leaves and lemon slices into ice cubes before serving the tea.

- **Vitamin C boost:** Lemons are high in vitamin C, an essential nutrient that boosts the immune system, supports skin health, and promotes collagen formation.

- **Calming effects:** Chamomile and mint can have mild calming effects, which may promote relaxation and help reduce stress or anxiety.

Point Value:

- **Weight Watchers Smart Points:** 0 points (if no added sweeteners are used).

Health Benefits:

- **Hydration:** Herbal iced tea helps with hydration, which is crucial for skin health, digestion, and overall energy levels.

- **Rich in antioxidants:** Depending on the type of herbal tea you use (especially green tea), it can be rich in antioxidants like polyphenols that help reduce oxidative stress.

- **Digestive aid:** Peppermint and chamomile are known for their soothing effects on the stomach, helping with digestion and relieving bloating or discomfort.

Freshly Squeezed Mediterranean Lemonade

Preparation Time: 10 minutes
Chill Time: 1 hour
Serving Unit: Serves 4-6

Ingredients:

- 4-5 large lemons (for about 1 cup fresh lemon juice)
- 1/4 cup honey, maple syrup, or sugar (adjust to taste)
- 4 cups cold water
- 1/2 teaspoon rosewater or orange blossom water (optional, for a floral twist)
- Ice cubes
- Lemon slices, for garnish
- Fresh mint or basil, for garnish

Procedure:

1. **Juice the lemons:**
   Cut the lemons in half and squeeze the juice into a pitcher, making sure to remove any seeds. You should have about 1 cup of fresh lemon juice.

2. **Sweeten the lemonade:**
   In a small saucepan, combine 1/4 cup of your preferred sweetener (honey, maple syrup, or sugar) with 1/4 cup of warm water. Stir until the sweetener dissolves completely. This will create a simple syrup that will blend well into your lemonade.

3. **Combine the lemonade:**
   Pour the fresh lemon juice into a large pitcher, then add the sweetened water. Add 4 cups of cold water to dilute the mixture to your desired strength, and stir well. Taste and adjust sweetness if needed.

4. **Optional floral twist:**
   For an extra touch of Mediterranean flavor, add 1/2 teaspoon of rosewater or orange blossom water to the lemonade. This adds a subtle floral fragrance and depth of flavor.

5. **Chill the lemonade:**
   Place the pitcher in the refrigerator and allow the lemonade to chill for at least 1 hour to meld the flavors and achieve a refreshing, cold drink.

6. **Serve:**
   To serve, pour the lemonade into glasses filled with ice. Garnish with fresh lemon slices and mint or basil leaves for a colorful and fragrant presentation.

7. **Enjoy:**
   Sip this revitalizing lemonade, perfect for hot summer days, gatherings, or as a delightful beverage with Mediterranean-inspired meals.

Nutritional Values (per serving):

- **Calories:** 35-50 kcal (depending on the sweetener used)

- **Protein:** 0g

- **Fat:** 0g

- **Carbohydrates:** 9-12g (from sweetener and lemons)

- **Fiber:** 0g

- **Sugar:** 8-12g (from honey, maple syrup, or sugar)

- **Sodium:** 5mg

Cooking Tips:

- **Adjust sweetness:** You can easily adjust the sweetness by adding more or less sweetener according to your taste preference.

- **Infuse herbs:** For a more complex flavor, try infusing the lemonade with fresh herbs such as basil, rosemary, or thyme. Simply add them to the pitcher before chilling and remove them before serving.

- **Lemon zest:** For a stronger lemon flavor, add a bit of lemon zest to the pitcher along with the juice. It will give the lemonade a more aromatic, citrusy punch.

- **Chill faster:** If you're in a rush, you can speed up the chilling process by placing the pitcher in the freezer for 20-30 minutes (but make sure not to freeze it!).

Point Value:

- **Weight Watchers Smart Points:** 1-2 points per serving (depending on the type and amount of sweetener used).

Health Benefits:

- **Vitamin C boost:** Lemons are an excellent source of vitamin C, which supports the immune system, boosts collagen production, and fights oxidative damage.

- **Hydration:** Lemonade is an excellent way to stay hydrated, especially during hot weather, promoting overall wellness and maintaining energy levels.

- **Detoxifying properties:** Lemons and honey are known for their detoxifying properties, helping cleanse the liver and digestive system.

- **Calming and refreshing:** Fresh mint and basil not only add flavor but can also have calming effects on the digestive system and reduce stress.

- **Supports digestion:** Lemon water (with or without the sweetness) is known to aid digestion, reduce bloating, and promote gut health.

Both of these refreshing drinks — the Herbal Iced Tea with Mint and Lemon and the Freshly Squeezed Mediterranean Lemonade — offer delightful, hydrating options for hot weather, gatherings, or just an afternoon pick-me-up. These beverages are simple to prepare, customizable to taste, and packed with beneficial nutrients from fresh herbs, citrus, and natural sweeteners. They provide a variety of health benefits, such as boosting hydration, improving digestion, and delivering antioxidant-rich ingredients that support overall well-being. Whether you choose the soothing, herbal flavors of mint and chamomile or the vibrant citrus burst of Mediterranean lemonade, both drinks are perfect for a healthy, flavorful alternative to sugary sodas or artificial beverages.

Conclusion

The Mediterranean diet is more than just a way of eating; it's a lifestyle. Inspired by the traditional eating patterns of countries bordering the Mediterranean Sea, such as Greece, Italy, Spain, and Southern France, this diet is rooted in fresh, seasonal, and minimally processed foods. It's celebrated for its numerous health benefits, including heart health, weight management, and even longevity.

The Mediterranean diet isn't a strict regimen, but rather a holistic approach to eating that prioritizes variety, balance, and wholesome, nutrient-dense foods. If you're looking to embrace this way of eating for better health, here's an in-depth look at the principles, benefits, and practical steps you can take to integrate it into your life.

Key Principles of the Mediterranean Diet

1. Focus on Plant-Based Foods

- **Fruits and Vegetables:** These should form the bulk of your diet. Aim to fill half of your plate with vegetables, fruits, or a combination of both at every meal. Choose a variety of colors to ensure you're getting a wide range of vitamins, minerals, and antioxidants.

- **Whole Grains:** Instead of refined grains, opt for whole grains like brown rice, quinoa, barley, farro, and whole wheat. These provide fiber, which supports digestive health and helps you feel full longer.

- **Legumes and Beans:** Beans, lentils, and peas are fantastic plant-based sources of protein and fiber. Incorporating them regularly can reduce your reliance on animal protein while also supporting heart health.

2. Healthy Fats

- **Olive Oil:** The cornerstone of the Mediterranean diet is olive oil, particularly extra virgin olive oil. It's rich in heart-healthy monounsaturated fats, which help reduce bad cholesterol and inflammation. Use it liberally for cooking, dressings, or drizzling over your dishes.

- **Nuts and Seeds:** Almonds, walnuts, pistachios, sunflower seeds, and flaxseeds are packed with healthy fats, protein, and fiber. They're also great sources of omega-3 fatty acids, which support brain and heart health.

- **Avocados:** While not native to the Mediterranean, avocados fit seamlessly into the diet due to their monounsaturated fats. They can be used in salads, dips, or even as a replacement for butter or cream.

3. Lean Proteins

- **Fish and Seafood:** Fish, especially fatty fishlike salmon, mackerel, sardines, and anchovies, should be eaten at least twice a week. These are rich in omega-3 fatty acids, which are crucial for reducing inflammation and supporting heart and brain health.

- **Poultry and Eggs:** While fish is the primary protein source, lean meats like chicken and turkey, as well as eggs, are consumed in moderation.

- **Dairy:** Greek yogurt, feta cheese, and other fermented dairy products are included in the Mediterranean diet. They offer a good source of protein, calcium, and probiotics for gut health.

4. Herbs and Spices

- The Mediterranean diet is known for its flavorful dishes, and this is achieved through the use of herbs and spices like garlic, basil, oregano, thyme, rosemary, mint, cumin, and paprika. These not only add vibrant flavors but also offer antioxidant and anti-inflammatory properties.

5. Moderate Wine Consumption

- In many Mediterranean cultures, wine, particularly red wine, is enjoyed in moderation with meals. It's believed that the polyphenols in wine (especially resveratrol) have cardiovascular benefits. The key is moderation—about 1 glass for women and 2 glasses for men per day.

6. Mindful Eating

- Meals are seen as an opportunity to enjoy food, socialize, and appreciate the sensory experience of eating. Meals tend to be leisurely, with time spent enjoying food with family and friends. This concept of mindful eating encourages people to savor each bite, which can help prevent overeating and promote healthier digestion.

Health Benefits of the Mediterranean Diet

1. Heart Health

- **Reduced Risk of Heart Disease:** The Mediterranean diet is renowned for its heart-healthy benefits. Numerous studies have shown that it can reduce the risk of heart disease, lower blood pressure, and improve cholesterol levels. The high intake of olive oil, nuts, and fish, all rich in omega-3s, plays a critical role in supporting cardiovascular health.

- **Anti-inflammatory Properties:** Chronic inflammation is linked to many diseases, including heart disease and arthritis. The Mediterranean diet's focus on antioxidant-rich foods—such as fruits, vegetables, olive oil, and fish—helps fight inflammation at the cellular level.

2. Weight Management

- **Sustainable Weight Loss:** The Mediterranean diet is not about restrictive calorie counting but rather about making healthier food choices. The high fiber content from whole grains, legumes, and vegetables helps keep you full for longer, while the healthy fats from olive oil, nuts, and seeds promote satiety without adding empty calories.

- **Improved Metabolism:** Regular consumption of lean proteins, fiber-rich foods, and healthy fats supports a balanced metabolism. Furthermore, the Mediterranean diet can help regulate insulin levels, which is beneficial for those managing blood sugar levels.

3. Longevity and Aging

- People in Mediterranean countries, particularly those in regions like Sardinia and Ikaria, are known for their longevity. Many of the residents in these regions live well into their 90s, and their diet is thought to play a major role in their extended lifespans. The Mediterranean diet's emphasis on antioxidants, healthy fats, and nutrient-dense foods contributes to overall health and longevity.

- **Brain Health:** The Mediterranean diet has been linked to a lower risk of cognitive decline and neurodegenerative diseases like Alzheimer's. The anti-inflammatory and antioxidant-rich foods, such as leafy greens, berries, fish, and olive oil, protect the brain and improve cognitive function.

4. Improved Digestion

- The diet's abundance of fiber from vegetables, fruits, whole grains, and legumes promotes healthy digestion and regular bowel movements. Additionally, fermented foods like yogurt and cheese provide beneficial probiotics that help maintain gut health.

5. Diabetes Prevention and Management

- Several studies show that the Mediterranean diet can reduce the risk of type 2 diabetes and improve blood sugar control in individuals who already have the condition. The combination of healthy fats, lean proteins, and whole grains helps regulate blood sugar levels, which is crucial for managing or preventing diabetes.

6. Mental Well-being

- There is growing evidence to suggest that the Mediterranean diet is not only beneficial for the body but also for the mind. The consumption of nutrient-dense, anti-inflammatory foods can have a positive effect on mood, reduce symptoms of depression and anxiety, and enhance cognitive function.

How to Embrace the Mediterranean Diet in Your Daily Life

1. Start with Simple Swaps

- **Olive Oil for Butter:** Begin by swapping out butter for extra virgin olive oil in cooking, dressings, and even for dipping bread.

- **Whole Grains Instead of Refined Carbs:** Choose whole grains like quinoa, barley, and brown rice over white rice, pasta, or bread. Whole grains are more nutritious and provide more fiber.

- **Add More Fish:** Aim for at least two servings of fatty fish per week, such as salmon, mackerel, or sardines. Try grilling, baking, or making fish tacos.

- **Snack on Nuts:** Instead of reaching for chips or processed snacks, try snacking on a handful of nuts, such as almonds or walnuts. These provide protein, healthy fats, and fiber.

2. Incorporate More Vegetables

- Aim to fill half your plate with vegetables at each meal. This could be in the form of salads, roasted vegetables, or vegetable-based dishes like ratatouille or stuffed peppers.

- Use herbs and spices to flavor your vegetables, making them more appealing and exciting to eat.

3. Enjoy Meals with Others

- One of the cornerstones of the Mediterranean way of life is enjoying meals with family and friends. Whether it's a simple dinner or a weekend barbecue, take the time to share your meals and enjoy the social connection that comes with eating together.

4. Stay Hydrated with Water and Herbal Teas

- Water is the drink of choice in the Mediterranean, with herbal teas like chamomile, mint, and fennel offering gentle ways to hydrate and support digestion.

- If you enjoy wine, have it in moderation, preferably with meals, and savor it for its complex flavors and aromas.

5. Practice Moderation

- The Mediterranean diet is not about extreme restriction or "cheat days." It's about balance. Enjoy all foods in moderation, including indulgent treats. The focus is on nutrient-dense foods, but there's always room for the occasional indulgence in sweets or a glass of wine.

Conclusion

The Mediterranean diet offers a refreshing, sustainable, and enjoyable approach to eating that not only promotes health but enhances your quality of life. By prioritizing whole, plant-based foods, healthy fats, and lean proteins, you can improve your heart health, manage your weight, reduce inflammation, and boost overall wellness.

Adopting the Mediterranean way of eating is a lifestyle choice that supports long-term health, mental well-being, and a joyful relationship with food. Whether you incorporate small changes or fully embrace the Mediterranean diet, every step towards eating more whole foods, enjoying meals with loved ones, and savoring every bite brings you closer to a healthier, more vibrant life.

Made in United States
Troutdale, OR
01/09/2025

27738796R00031